Keto C

# Cookbook

## For Beginners

A Simple Guide With 40 Quick And Easy Recipes For Boost Your Metabolism And Live Healthy.

## Carol Gervais

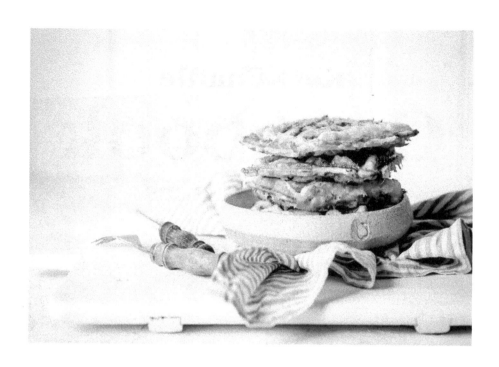

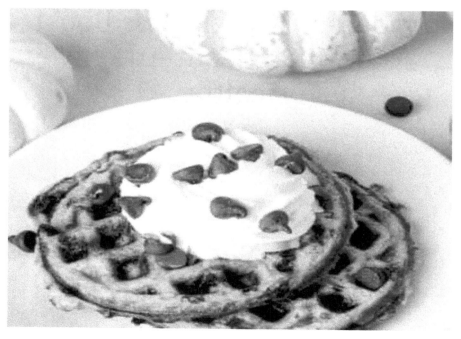

# TABLE OF CONTENTS

# INTRODUCTION

K eto Diet is a high-fat, low-carb diet that is an increasingly popular way to lose weight. Keto is short for "ketosis", which occurs when the body has depleted its sugar stores, so it burns stored fat instead of glucose in order to produce energy.

Losing weight on a keto diet sounds pretty easy; just eat a few bacon sandwiches and you'll be slimmer in no time. However, there are drawbacks to this diet, including very low levels of vegetables and fruit (so important for fiber and other nutrients) as well as constipation from lack of dietary fiber. Here are some tips:

- It's important to drink plenty of water, not only because you may be eating more sodium than you need, but because staying hydrated will help your body process proteins and fats more efficiently.

- For best results, stay away from most fruits and vegetables. Some berries are allowed; others aren't. Vegetables that are considered "low in carbs" or "leafy greens" are fine—but there is a difference between low-carb and high-fiber. As a rule of thumb, if it looks like it has the texture of tree bark or is covered with seeds or bulbs (e.g., artichokes), it probably has a lot of carbs and should be avoided.

- Be careful with spices, which tend to have a lot of sugar; salt is OK. It can be easy to go overboard on spices.

- Eat plenty of salmon, tuna and egg whites. Meat—including beef, chicken, pork and lamb—should comprise 20 to 25 percent of your total diet. (Be aware that "lean" meat is often not very lean. Be prepared to trim off most of that fat before cooking.) A little bacon or sausage is fine, too.

- Avoid condiments and sauces, including barbecue sauce and ketchup. These are full of sugar and other unhealthy ingredients.

- Drink mostly water (or unsweetened drinks such as tea or coffee). Try to avoid drinks with a lot of added sugar, like fruit juice or alcohol. If you choose to drink wine, go for the dry stuff—red wine is best.

Now, for Chaffles.

What is Chaffle?

Keto chaffle recipe is a versatile and easy-to-make low carb pancake that only requires 2 ingredients. It's a way to satisfy your sweet cravings while staying keto!

Chaffle is made from cheese and eggs. You will need grated cheddar cheese (use any kind of cheese you have on hand) and eggs, beaten together, then fried in a pan with butter or coconut oil.

Chaffles are perfect for a low carb breakfast, lunch or dinner and can be a treat right out of the pan, with butter!

Why Keto and Chaffle is a perfect combination?

Keto Chaffle is a great way to satisfy your sweet cravings while staying 100% in ketosis. It helps you feel fuller for longer but at the same time it's not a high carb treat.

Chaffle gives you a lot of energy and it's an easy way to prepare breakfast if you want it to be ready quickly when you get up or even if you're in a hurry so it can be prepared on the go without any issues.

Keto Chaffle tastes amazing plain, with butter or with any toppings you like and it can also be used as sandwich bread substitute.

# KETOGENIC DIET AND ITS BENEFITS

## What is Ketogenic Diet?

The ketogenic diet is a low-carb, high-fat diet. This means that the macronutrient ratio of your diet should consist mainly of fat and protein with only a small percentage of carbohydrates.

The idea behind the ketogenic diet is to force your body to use fat rather than glucose as its primary fuel source. When we are in ketosis, we can function on almost any fuel source.

## Benefits of the Ketogenic Diet

The benefits of the ketogenic diet are as follows:

1. No need to count calories.

On this diet, you can eat as much as you want. Since there are no grains, the carbohydrates in the diet are very low, and so you will not take in many calories.

2. There is no need to spend a lot of money on expensive foods.

Since this diet is high in fat, one of the cheapest sources of fat is chicken thighs and legs and other skinless poultry parts or meats from around the animal, such as organ meats (heart, liver, etc.).

3. Low levels of Beta-hydroxybutyrate (ketone body) is suitable for brain health

The ketogenic diet can increase the level of ketone bodies by 10 times than normal dietary levels through fat metabolism.

4. Decreased risk of heart disease

Many people can lower their LDL (bad) cholesterol by 75-90% and triglyceride levels by 60%.

5. Less inflammation

Because there are no carbohydrates in the ketogenic diet, your body becomes very efficient at burning ketones as fuel. This is excellent news if you have an autoimmune disorder like rheumatoid arthritis or Crohn's disease because inflammation is often linked to autoimmune problems.

6. Fast weight loss

People usually start losing weight within two weeks of starting the diet.

7. Increased energy levels

The ketogenic diet can increase your energy levels because you will be consuming a high-fat diet with very few carbohydrates.

8. No constant hunger

When people are on a ketogenic diet, they are in "ketosis." This means that their bodies are using fat as an almost complete fuel source. This is the opposite of how most people function in a non-ketogenic state, which usually involves using carbohydrates (sugars) as a practically whole fuel source. Because the ketogenic diet is so different, the body is forced to use fat as its primary fuel source to function. This means you won't be hungry all the time once you get the hang of it.

9. No need for cheat meals

Since carbohydrates are reduced in this diet, cheating on the ketogenic diet will not help you lose weight because your body does not have carbohydrates stored to keep your metabolism running, being that fat is used instead of sugar/carbs.

10. No need to buy expensive supplements

Since the diet is not very restrictive, you won't need to buy many supplements besides vitamin D3 if you are deficient.

11. You can gain muscle and lose fat at the same time

When you do strength training with a ketogenic diet, the weight loss is due to body fat (adipose tissue), not muscle mass. Many people find it difficult to lose weight because they are losing muscle mass and body fat, which is not suitable for overall health. However, because this diet encourages protein consumption at every meal, as well as healthy fats, your amino acid intake will be sufficient to preserve your muscles without inhibiting your weight loss.

## Foods Allowed

Here is the list of foods you can eat during the ketogenic diet:

1.  Meat, poultry, fish, shellfish, and eggs from pasture-fed animals (animals are fed a grass-fed diet)
2.  Fish and seafood caught in the wild
3.  Eggs from pastured hens
4.  Vegetables, including root vegetables such as beets and carrots and leafy greens such as spinach and kale.

5. Healthy fats such as coconut oil or olive oil that can be used in place of butter or other oils (11 grams per day maximum)

6. Nuts and seeds such as macadamia nuts, walnuts, and pumpkin seeds

7. Low to moderate amounts of dairy products such as yogurt and cheese

8. Non-starchy vegetables such as broccoli, cauliflower, and other cruciferous vegetables

9. Fruits

## Foods That Are Not Allowed

Foods that are not allowed

When following the keto diet, you will want to avoid eating the following foods:

1. Grains including wheat, oats, rice, and corn

2. Sugar, including honey, maple syrup, and sugar in all its forms

3. Vegetable oils such as canola, sunflower, and soybean oil

4. Trans fats such as margarine and vegetable shortening

5. Juices and sugary drinks such as soda, fruit juices with added sugar or artificial sweeteners, or milk alternatives made with grains such as almond milk

6. Grain-based dairy products such as butter and yogurt

7. Legumes such as beans, soybeans, and peanuts

8. Starchy vegetables such as potatoes, peas, and corn

9. Processed foods of any kind, including sauces and any food that contains a high percentage of preservatives

10. Beer (pure alcohol)

11. Low-fat or nonfat dairy products such as yogurt and cheese (dairy products that are low in fat but have carbohydrates)

12. Fruit juices with added sugars or artificial sweeteners

# Volume (liquid)

| US Customary | Metric |
|---|---|
| 1/8 teaspoon | .6 ml |
| 1/4 teaspoon | 1.2 ml |
| 1/2 teaspoon | 2.5 ml |
| 3/4 teaspoon | 3.7 ml |
| 1 teaspoon | 5 ml |
| 1 tablespoon | 15 ml |
| 2 tablespoon or 1 fluid ounce | 30 ml |
| 1/4 cup or 2 fluid ounces | 59 ml |
| 1/3 cup | 79 ml |
| 1/2 cup | 118 ml |
| 2/3 cup | 158 ml |
| 3/4 cup | 177 ml |
| 1 cup or 8 fluid ounces | 237 ml |
| 2 cups or 1 pint | 473 ml |
| 4 cups or 1 quart | 946 ml |
| 8 cups or 1/2 gallon | 1.9 liters |
| 1 gallon | 3.8 liters |

# Weight (mass)

| US contemporary (ounces) | Metric (grams) |
| --- | --- |
| 1/2 ounce | 14 grams |
| 1 ounce | 28 grams |
| 3 ounces | 85 grams |
| 3.53 ounces | 100 grams |
| 4 ounces | 113 grams |
| 8 ounces | 227 grams |
| 12 ounces | 340 grams |
| 16 ounces or 1 pound | 454 grams |

# Volume Equivalents (liquid)*

| 3 teaspoons | 1 tablespoon | 0.5 fluid ounce |
| --- | --- | --- |
| 2 tablespoons | 1/8 cup | 1 fluid ounce |
| 4 tablespoons | 1/4 cup | 2 fluid ounces |
| 5 1/3 tablespoons | 1/3 cup | 2.7 fluid ounces |
| 8 tablespoons | 1/2 cup | 4 fluid ounces |
| 12 tablespoons | 3/4 cup | 6 fluid ounces |
| 16 tablespoons | 1 cup | 8 fluid ounces |
| 2 cups | 1 pint | 16 fluid ounces |

# BREAKFAST CHAFFLE RECIPES

## 1. Cinnamon Swirls Chaffle

**Preparation Time:** 12 minutes

**Cooking Time:** 6 minutes

Serving: 2

**Ingredients:**

Icing

- Butter: 2 tablespoons unsalted butter
- Cream cheese: 2 oz. softened
- Vanilla: 1 teaspoon
- Splenda: 2 tablespoons

Chaffle

- Egg: 2
- Almond flour: 2 tablespoons
- Cinnamon: 2 teaspoons
- Splenda: 2 tablespoons
- Cream Cheese: 2 oz. softened
- Vanilla Extract: 2 teaspoons
- Vanilla extract: 2 teaspoons

Cinnamon Drizzle

- Splenda: 2 tablespoons
- Cinnamon: 2 teaspoons
- Butter: 1 tablespoon

## Directions:

1. Preheat and grease a waffle maker. a combined mixture of all ingredients, evenly mixed and pour into the waffle maker.
2. Cooking for 4 minutes till chaffles turns crispy, and then set aside. Using a mixing bowl, a mix of all ingredients for icing and the cinnamon drizzle, then heat using a microwave for 12 seconds to soften. Pour heated icing and cinnamon on the cool chaffles to enjoy.

## Nutrition:

- Calories 134 Kcal
- Fat: 13.1 g
- Protein: 2.2 g
- Net carb: 1.1 g

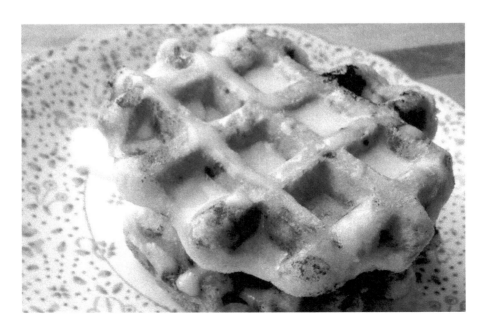

## 2. Japanese Styled Chaffle

**Preparation Time:** 12 minutes

**Cooking Time:** 6 minutes

**Servings:** 2

**Ingredients:**

- Egg: 1
- Bacon: 1 slice
- Green onion: 1 stalk
- Mozzarella cheese: 1/2 cup (shredded)
- Kewpie Mayo: 2 tablespoons

**Directions:**

1. Preheat and grease the waffle maker. Using a mixing bowl, a mix containing kewpie mayo with beaten egg, then add in ½ chopped green onion with the other ½ kept aside, and ¼ inches of cut bacon into the mixture.
2. Mix evenly. Sprinkle the base of the waffle maker with 1/8 cup of shredded Mozzarella and pour in the mixture, then top with more shredded mozzarella. With a closed lid, heat the waffle for 5 minutes to a crunch and then remove the chaffle and allow cooking for a few minutes.
3. Repeat for the remaining chaffles mixture to make more batter. Serve by garnishing the chaffle with the leftover chopped green onions. Enjoy.

**Nutrition:**

- Calories 92 Kcal
- Fat: 7 g
- Protein: 1 g
- Net carb: 2 g

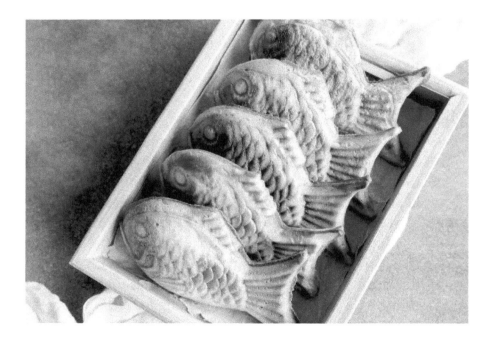

# 3. Keto Strawberry Chaffle

**Preparation Time:** 10 minutes

**Cooking Time:** 5 minutes

**Servings:** 2

**Ingredient**

1. 1 egg
2. 1/4 cup Mozzarella cheese
3. 1 tablespoonful cream cheese
4. 1/4 teaspoonful baking powder
5. 2 sliced strawberries
6. 1 teaspoonful strawberry extract

**Directions:**

1. Preheat waffle maker.
2. In a little bowl, beat the egg.
3. Add the rest of the ingredients.
4. The waffle maker is sprayed with nonstick cooking spray.
5. Divide the mix into two equal parts.
6. Cooking a portion of the mix for around 4 minutes or until golden brown colored.

## Nutrition:

- Calories: 249
- Fat: 20g
- Carbs: 3g
- Protein: 15g

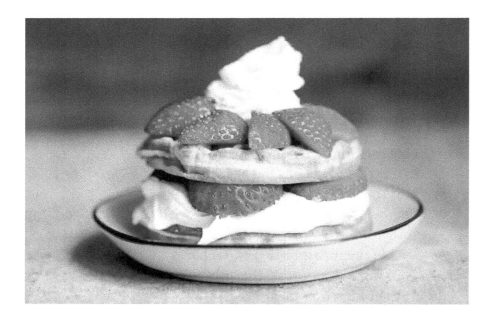

# 4. Keto Crunchy Chaffle

**Preparation Time:** 15 minutes

**Cooking Time:** 8 minutes

**Servings:** 2

**Ingredients:**

- 2 Large Eggs
- 1/2 Cup Shredded Mozzarella cheese (pressed firmly)
- 1/2 teaspoon Baking Powder
- 1 Tablespoon Erythritol (powder), or sweetener (however powder is most ideal)
- 1/2 teaspoon Vanilla Extract

**Directions:**

1. Heat You Waffle Iron on the high heat setting. I used a 7-inch waffle Iron and this formula fits nicely for one huge waffle. If you have a smaller waffle iron, you will need to divide the recipe into two waffles.
2. Put all ingredients into a Bullet or a Blender and blend for 10 seconds.
3. Pour the mix into a very hot and dry waffle Iron. It will look thin once poured but have no fear it significantly increases in size when it cooking (and you'll need to keep an eye on it to avoid overflow when cooking!). Let the waffle to Cooking for 3-4 minutes or much more! The waffle is done once the entire waffle is golden dark-colored, which takes longer than a normal waffle would. You can use a fork to flip your waffle to ensure that each side has even colors if it doesn't look done after some time. Let waffle cool for 3-4 minutes before eating since it may become brown on cooling

4. Serve with gobs of grass-fed butter and sugar-free syrup, or whatever topping you want.

## Nutrition:

- Calories: 155
- Fat: 14g
- Protein: 5g
- Net Carbs: 2g

# 5. Keto Silver Dollar Pancakes

**Preparation Time:** 10 minutes

**Cooking Time:** 5 minutes

**Servings:** 2

## Ingredients

- (3) Eggs
- 1/2 Cup (105 G) Cottage Cheese
- 1/3 Cup (37.33 G) Superfine Almond Flour
- 1/4 Cup (62.5 G) Unsweetened Almond Milk
- 2 Tablespoons Truvia

Vanilla Extract

- 1 Teaspoon Baking Powder
- Cooking Oil Spray

## Directions:

1. place ingredients in a blender in the order listed above. Mix until you have a smooth, fluid batter.
2. Heat a nonstick pan on medium-high temperature. Spray with oil or margarine.
3. Place 2 tablespoons of batter at once to make little, dollar hotcakes. This is an extremely fluid, sensitive batter so don't
4. attempt to make big pancakes with this one as they won't flip over easily.
5. Cooking every pancake until the top of the hotcake has made little air pockets and the air pockets have vanished, around 1-2 minutes.
6. Using a spatula, tenderly loosen the pan cake, and afterward flip over.
7. Make the remainder of the pancakes and serve hot.

## Nutrition:

- Calories: 110
- Fat: 8g
- Protein: 2g
- Net Carbs: 7g

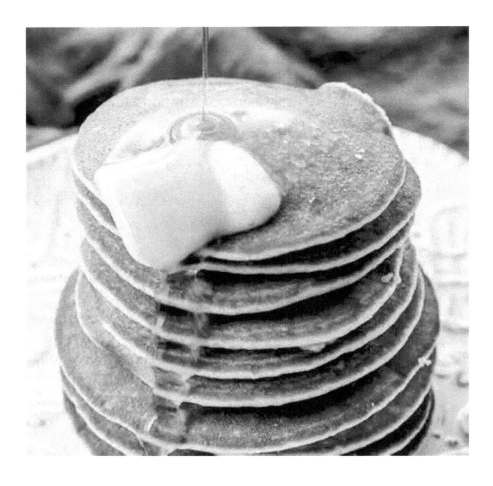

# 6. Keto Chaffle Waffle

**Preparation Time:** 10 minutes

**Cooking Time:** 6 minutes

**Servings:** 2

**Ingredients:**

- 1 egg
- ½ cup of shredded Mozzarella cheese
- 1 ½ table-spoon of almond flour
- Pinch of baking powder

**Directions:**

1. Start by turning your waffle maker on and preheating it. During the time of pre-heating, in a bowl, whisk the egg and shredded Mozzarella cheese together. If you do not have shredded Mozzarella cheese, you can use the shredder to shred your cheese, then add the almond powder and baking powder to the bowl and whisk them until the mixture is consistent.
2. Then pour the mixture onto the waffle machine. Make sure you pour it to the center of the mixture will come out of the edges on closing the machine. Close the machine and let the waffles cooking until golden brown. Then you can serve your tasty chaffle waffles.

**Nutrition:**

- Calories: 170
- Fat: 15g
- Protein: 7g
- Net Carbs: 2g

## 7. Keto Chaffle Topped with Salted Caramel Syrup

**Preparation Time:** 15 minutes

**Cooking Time:** 10 minutes

**Servings:** 2

**Ingredients:**

- 1 egg
- ½ cup of Mozzarella cheese
- ¼ cup of cream
- 2 tablespoon of collagen powder
- 1 ½ tablespoon of almond flour
- 1 ½ tablespoon of unsalted butter
- Pinch of salt
- ¾ tablespoon of powdered erythritol
- Pinch of baking powder

**Directions:**

1. Begin by preheating your waffle machine by switching it on and turning the heat to medium. Whisk together the chaffle ingredients that include the egg, Mozzarella cheese, almond flour, and baking powder. Pour the mixture on the waffle machine. Let it cooking until golden brown. You can make up to two chaffles with this method.

2. To make the caramel syrup, you will need to turn on the flame under a pan to medium heat Melt the unsalted butter on the pan. Then turn the heat low and add collagen powder and erythritol to the pan and whisk them. Gradually add the cream and remove from heat.

Then add the salt and continue to whisk. Pour the syrup onto the chaffle, and here you go.

## Nutrition:

- Calories: 75
- Fat: 7g
- Protein: 1g
- Net Carbs: 3g

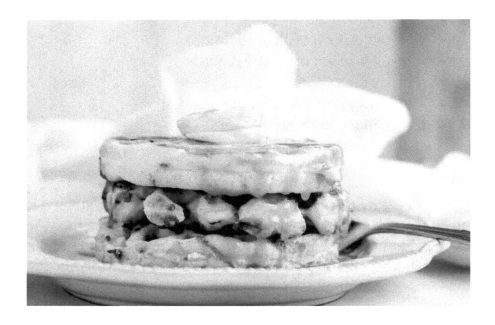

# 8. Keto Chaffle Bacon Sandwich

**Preparation Time:** 15 minutes

**Cooking Time:** 10 minutes

**Servings:** 2

**Ingredients**:

- 1 egg
- ½ cup of shredded Mozzarella cheese
- 2 Tablespoon of coconut flour
- 2 strips of pork or beef bacon
- 1 slice of any type of cheese
- 2 tablespoon of coconut oil

## Directions:

1. To make the chaffle, you will be following the typical recipe for making a chaffle. Start by warming your waffle machine to medium heat. In a bowl, beat 1 egg, ½ cup of Mozzarella cheese, and almond flour. Pour the mixture on the waffle machine. Let it cooking until it is golden brown. Then remove in a plate.
2. Warm coconut oil in a pan over medium heat. Then place the bacon strips in the pan. Cooking until crispy over medium heat. Assemble the bacon and cheese on the chaffle.

**Nutrition:**

- Calories: 225
- Fat: 19g
- Protein: 8g
- Net Carbs: 3g

# BASIC SANDWICH AND CAKE CHAFFLE RECIPES

## 9. Keto Chocolate Waffle Cake

**Preparation Time:** 5 minutes

**Cooking Time:** 5 minutes

**Servings:** 3

**Ingredients:**

- 2 tbs cocoa
- 2 tbs monkfruit confectioner's
- 1 egg
- 1/4 teaspoon baking powder
- 1 tbs heavy whipped cream
- Frosted ingredients
- 2 tbs monkfruit confectioners
- 2 tbs cream cheese softens, room temperature
- 1/4 teaspoon transparent vanilla

**Directions:**

1. Whip the egg in a small bowl.
2. Add the rest of the ingredients and mix well until smooth and creamy.
3. Pour half of the batter into a mini waffle maker and cooking until fully cooked for 2 1/2 to 3 minutes.
4. Add the sweetener, cream cheese, and vanilla in a separate small bowl. Mix the frosting until all is well embedded.
5. Spread the frosting on the cake after it has cooled down to room temperature.

**Nutrition:**

- Calories: 352.3
- Protein: 20 g
- Carbohydrates: 41.2 g
- Fats: 12 g

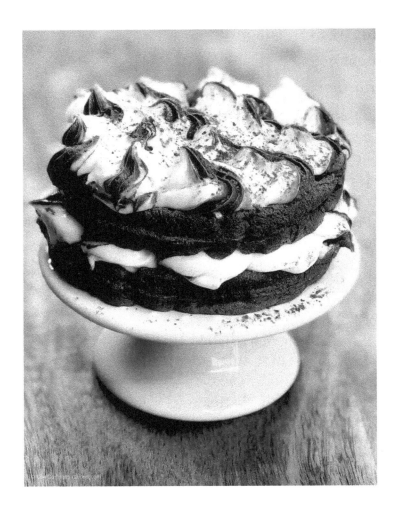

## 10. Keto Vanilla Twinkie Copycat Chaffle

**Preparation Time:** 5 minutes

**Cooking Time:** 4 minutes

**Servings:** 4

**Ingredients:**

- 2 tablespoons of butter (cooled)
- 2 oz. cream cheese softened
- Two large egg room temperature
- 1 teaspoon of vanilla essence
- Optional 1/2 teaspoon vanilla cupcake extract
- 1/4 cup lacanto confectionery
- Pinch of salt
- 1/4 cup almond flour
- 2 tablespoons coconut powder
- 1 teaspoon baking powder

**Directions:**

1. Preheat corndog maker.
2. Melt the butter and let cool for 1 minute.
3. Whisk the butter until the eggs are creamy.
4. Add vanilla, extract, sweetener and salt and mix well.
5. Add almond flour, coconut flour, baking powder.
6. Mix until well incorporated.
7. Add ~ 2 tbs batter to each well and spread evenly.
8. Close and lock the lid and cooking for 4 minutes.
9. Remove and cool the rack.

**Nutrition:**

- Calories: 290
- Fats: 10 g
- Carbohydrates: 13 g
- Protein: 38 g

# 11.  Carrot Cake Chaffles

**Preparation Time:** 5 minutes

**Cooking Time:** 5 minutes

**Servings:** 6

**Ingredients:**

- 1/2 cup chopped carrot
- 1 egg
- 2 t butter melted
- 2 t heavy whipped cream
- 3/4 cup almond flour
- 1 walnut chopped
- 2 t powder sweetener
- 2 tsp. cinnamon
- 1 tsp. pumpkin spice
- 1 tsp. baking powder
- Cream cheese frosting
- 4 oz. cream cheese softened
- 1/4 cup powdered sweetener
- 1 teaspoon of vanilla essence
- 1-2 t heavy whipped cream according to your preferred consistency

**Directions:**

1. Mix dry ingredients such as almond flour, cinnamon, pumpkin spices, baking powder, powdered sweeteners, and walnut pieces.
2. Add the grated carrots, eggs, melted butter and cream.
3. Add a 3t batter to a preheated mini waffle maker. Cooking for 2 1 / 2-3 minutes.

4. Mix the frosted ingredients with a hand mixer with a whisk until well mixed
5. Stack waffles and add a frost between each layer!

**Nutrition:**

- Calories: 400
- Carbohydrates: 11 g
- Protein: 44 g
- Fats: 20 g

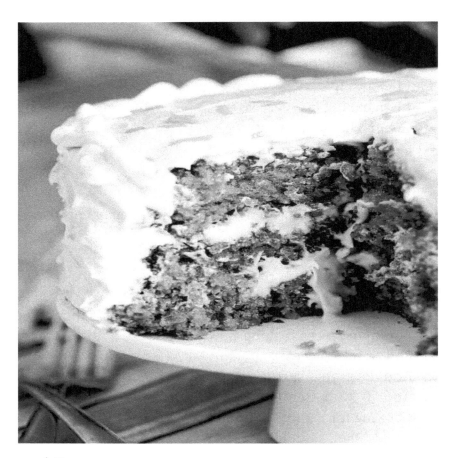

## 12. Easy Soft Cinnamon Rolls Chaffle Cake

**Preparation Time:** 5 minutes

**Cooking Time:** 12 minutes

**Servings:** 3

**Ingredients:**

- 1 egg
- 1/2 cup Mozzarella cheese
- 1/2 tsp. vanilla
- 1/2 tsp. cinnamon
- 1 tbs monk fruit confectioner's blend

**Directions:**

1. Put the eggs in a small bowl.
2. Add the remaining ingredients.
3. Spray to the waffle maker with a non-stick cooking spray.
4. Make two chaffles.
5. Separate the mixture.
6. Cooking half of the mixture for about 4 minutes or until golden.
7. Notes added glaze: 1 tb of cream cheese melted in a microwave for 15 seconds, and 1 tb of monk fruit confectioners mix. Mix it and spread it over the moist fabric.
8. Additional frosting: 1 tb cream cheese (high temp), 1 tb room temp butter (low temp) and 1 tb monk fruit confectioners' mix. Mix all the ingredients together and spread to the top of the cloth.
9. Top with optional frosting, glaze, nuts, sugar-free syrup, whipped cream or simply dust with monk fruit sweets.

**Nutrition:**

- Calories: 320
- Fats: 10 g
- Carbohydrates: 15 g
- Protein: 45 g

# 13. Banana Pudding Chaffle Cake

**Preparation Time:** 5 minutes

**Cooking Time:** 5 minutes

**Servings:** 2

**Ingredients:**

- 1 large egg yolk
- 1/2 cup fresh cream
- 3 t powder sweetener
- 1 / 4-1 / 2 teaspoon xanthan gum
- 1/2 teaspoon banana extract

Banana chaffle ingredients

- 1 oz. softened cream cheese
- 1/4 cup Mozzarella cheese shredded
- 1 egg
- 1 teaspoon banana extract
- 2 t sweetener
- 1 tsp. baking powder
- 4 t almond flour

**Directions:**

1. Mix heavy cream, powdered sweetener and egg yolk in a small pot. Whisk constantly until the sweetener has dissolved and the mixture is thick.
2. Cooking for 1 minute. Add xanthan gum and whisk.
3. Remove from heat, add a pinch of salt and banana extract and stir well.
4. Transfer to a glass dish and cover the pudding with plastic wrap. Refrigerate.
5. Mix all ingredients together. Cooking in a preheated mini waffle maker.

## Nutrition:

- Calories: 478
- Protein: 30 g
- Carbohydrates: 22 g
- Fats: 29 g

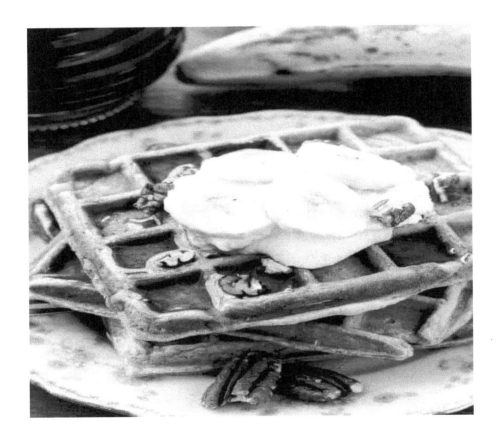

# 14.  Keto Cake

**Preparation Time:** 5 minutes

**Cooking Time:** 5 minutes

**Servings:** 2

**Ingredients:**

- 2 tbs sugar free peanut butter powder
- 2 tbs monkfruit confectioner 's
- 1 egg
- 1/4 teaspoon baking powder
- 1 tbs heavy whipped cream
- 1/4 teaspoon peanut butter extract
- Peanut butter frosting ingredients
- 2 tbs monkfruit confectioners
- 1 tbs butter softens, room temperature
- 1 tbs unsweetened natural peanut butter or peanut butter powder
- 2 tbs cream cheese softens, room temperature
- 1/4 tsp. vanilla

**Directions:**

1. Serve the eggs in a small bowl.
2. Add the remaining ingredients and mix well until the dough is smooth and creamy.
3. If you don't have peanut butter extract, you can skip it. It adds absolutely wonderful, more powerful peanut butter flavor and is worth investing in this extract.
4. Pour half of the butter into a mini waffle maker and cooking for 2-3 minutes until it is completely cooked.

5. In another small bowl, add sweetener, cream cheese, sugar-free natural peanut butter and vanilla. Mix frosting until everything is well incorporated.
6. When the waffle cake has completely cooled to room temperature, spread the frosting.
7. Or you can even pipe the frost!
8. Or you can heat the frosting and add 1/2 teaspoon of water to make the peanut butter are pill and drizzle chaffle. I like it anyway!

**Nutrition:**
- Calories: 117
- Protein: 14 g
- Carbohydrates: 2.2 g
- Fats: 7 g

## 15. Keto Italian Cream Chaffle Cake

**Preparation Time:** 5 minutes

**Cooking Time:** 3 minutes

**Servings:** 1

**Ingredients:**

For sweet chaffle:

- 4 oz. cream cheese softens, room temperature
- 4 eggs
- 1 tablespoon butter
- 1 teaspoon of vanilla essence
- 1/2 teaspoon of cinnamon
- 1 tbsp. monk fruit sweetener or favorite keto approved sweetener
- 4 tablespoons coconut powder
- 1 tablespoon almond flour
- 1 1/2 cup baking powder
- 1 tablespoon coconut
- 1 walnut chopped

Italian cream frosting ingredients

- 2 oz. Cream cheese softens, room temperature
- 2 cups of butter room temp
- 2 tbs monk fruit sweetener or favorite keto approved sweetener
- 1/2 teaspoon vanilla

**Directions:**

1. In a medium blender, add cream cheese, eggs, melted butter, vanilla, sweeteners, coconut flour, almond flour, and baking powder. Optional: add shredded coconut and

walnut to the mixture or save for matting. Both methods are great!

2. Mix the ingredients high until smooth and creamy.
3. Preheat mini waffle maker.
4. Add ingredients to the preheated waffle maker.
5. Cooking for about 2-3 minutes until the waffle is complete.
6. Remove chaffle and let cool.
7. In a separate bowl, add all the ingredients together and start frosting. Stir until smooth and creamy.
8. When the chaffle has cooled completely, frost the cake.
9. Note: Create 8 mini chaffles or 3-4 large chaffles.

**Nutrition:**

- Calories: 98
- Fat: 0.7g
- Carbs: 19.2g
- Protein: 3.8g
- Fiber: 3.4g

# 16. Keto Boston Cream Pie Chaffle Cake

**Preparation Time:** 10 minutes

**Cooking Time:** 5 minutes

**Servings:** 4

**Ingredients:**

Ingredients for chaffle cake:

- 2 eggs
- 1/4 cup almond flour
- Coconut flower 1 teaspoon
- 2 tablespoons of melted butter
- 2 tablespoons of cream cheese
- 20 drops of Boston cream extract
- 1/2 teaspoon of vanilla essence
- 1/2 teaspoon baking powder
- 2 tablespoons sweetener or monk fruit
- 1/4 teaspoon xanthan powder
- Custard ingredients
- 1/2 cup fresh cream
- 1/2 teaspoon of vanilla essence
- 1/2 tbs swerve confectioner's sweetener
- 2 yolks
- 1/8 teaspoon xanthan gum

Ingredients for ganache:

- 2 tbs heavy whipped cream
- 2 tbs unsweetened baking chocolate bar chopped
- 1 tbs swerve confectioners' sweetener

## Directions:

1. Preheat the mini waffle iron to render the cake chops first.
2. In a mixer, mix all the ingredients of the cake and blend until smooth and fluffy. It's only supposed to take a few minutes.
3. Heat the heavy whipping cream to a boil on the stovetop. While it's dry, whisk the egg yolks together in a small separate dish.
4. Once the cream is boiling, add half of it to the egg yolks. Make sure you're whisking it together while you're slowly pouring it into the mixture.
5. Add the egg and milk mixture to the rest of the cream in the stovetop pan and stir vigorously for another 2-3 minutes.
6. Take the custard off the heat and whisk in your vanilla and xanthan gum. Then set aside to cool and thicken.
7. Place the ganache ingredients in a small bowl. Microwave for about 20 seconds, stir. Repeat, if necessary. Careful not to overheat and roast the ganache. Just do it 20 seconds at a time until it's completely melted.
8. Assemble and enjoy your Boston cream pie chaffle cake!

## Nutrition:

- Calories: 105
- Fat: 1.1g
- Carbs: 18.3g
- Protein: 5.4g
- Fiber: 4.9g

# SAVORY CHAFFLE RECIPES

## 17.  Parmesan Garlic Chaffle

**Preparation Time:** 6 minutes

**Cooking Time:** 5 Minutes

**Servings:** 2

**Ingredients:**

- 1 Tbsp fresh garlic minced
- 2 Tbsp butter
- 1-oz cream cheese, cubed
- 2 Tbsp almond flour
- 1 tsp baking soda
- 2 large eggs
- 1 tsp dried chives
- ½ cup parmesan cheese, shredded
- ¾ cup mozzarella cheese, shredded

**Directions:**

1. Heat cream cheese and butter in a saucepan over medium-low until melted.
2. Add garlic and cook, stirring, for minutes.
3. Turn on waffle maker to heat and oil it with cooking spray.
4. In a small mixing bowl, whisk together flour and baking soda, then set aside.
5. In a separate bowl, beat eggs for 1 minute 30 seconds on high, then add in cream cheese mixture and beat for 60 seconds more.

6. Add flour mixture, chives, and cheeses to the bowl and stir well.
7. Add ¼ cup batter to waffle maker.
8. Close and cook for 4 minutes, until golden brown.
9. Repeat for remaining batter.
10. Add favorite toppings and serve.

## Nutrition:

- Calories: 236
- Total Fat: 23g
- Protein: 6g
- Total Carbs: 5g
- Fiber: 3g
- Net Carbs: 2g
- Cholesterol: 0mg

# 18. Chicken & Veggies Chaffles

**Preparation Time:** 10 minutes

**Cooking Time:** 15 Minutes

**Servings:** 2

**Ingredients:**

- 1/3 cup cooked grass-fed chicken, chopped
- 1/3 cup cooked spinach, chopped
- 1/3 cup marinated artichokes, chopped
- 1 organic egg, beaten
- 1/3 cup Mozzarella cheese, shredded
- 1 ounce cream cheese, softened
- ¼ teaspoon garlic powder

**Directions:**

1. Preheat a mini waffle iron and then grease it.
2. In a medium bowl, place all ingredients and mix until well combined.
3. Place 1/of the mixture into preheated waffle iron and cook for about 4-5 minutes or until golden brown.
4. Repeat with the remaining mixture.
5. Serve warm.

## Nutrition:

- Calories: 227
- Total Fat: 19g
- Protein: 10g
- Total Carbs: 8g
- Fiber: 4g
- Net Carbs: 4g
- Cholesterol: 143mg

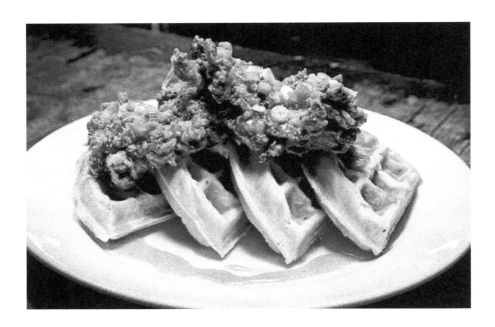

## 19. Turkey Chaffles

**Preparation Time:** 10 minutes

**Cooking Time:** 16 Minutes

**Servings:** 2

**Ingredients:**

- ½ cup cooked turkey meat, chopped
- 2 organic eggs, beaten
- ½ cup Parmesan cheese, grated
- ½ cup Mozzarella, shredded
- ¼ teaspoon poultry seasoning
- ¼ teaspoon onion powder

**Directions:**

1. Preheat a mini waffle iron and then grease it.
2. In a medium bowl, place all ingredients and mix until well combined.
3. Place ¼ of the mixture into preheated waffle iron and cook for about 4 minutes or until golden brown.
4. Repeat with the remaining mixture.
5. Serve warm.

## Nutrition:

- Calories: 365
- Total Fat: 33g
- Protein: 14g
- Total Carbs: 10g
- Fiber: 6g
- Net Carbs: 4g
- Cholesterol: 0mg

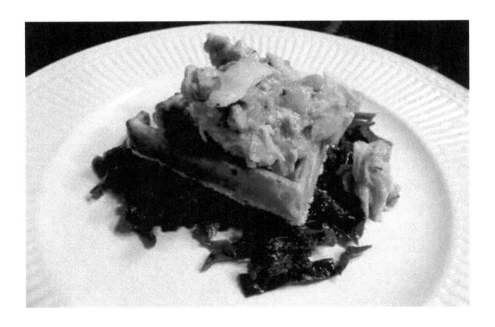

# 20. Chicken & Zucchini Chaffles

**Preparation Time:** 10 minutes

**Cooking Time:** 5 Minutes

**Servings:** 9

**Ingredients:**

- 4 ounces cooked grass-fed chicken, chopped
- 2 cups zucchini, shredded and squeezed
- ¼ cup scallion, chopped
- 2 large organic eggs
- ½ cup Mozzarella cheese, shredded
- ½ cup Cheddar cheese, shredded
- ½ cup blanched almond flour
- 1 teaspoon organic baking powder
- ½ teaspoon garlic salt
- ½ teaspoon onion powder

**Directions:**

1. Preheat a waffle iron and then grease it.
2. In a medium bowl, place all ingredients and mix until well combined.
3. Divide the mixture into 9 portions.
4. Place 1 portion of the mixture into preheated waffle iron and cook for about 2-3 minutes or until golden brown.
5. Repeat with the remaining mixture.
6. Serve warm.

**Nutrition:**

- Calories: 292
- Total Fat: 26g
- Protein: 10g
- Total Carbs: 9g
- Fiber: 2g
- Net Carbs: 7g
- Cholesterol: 0mg

## 21.    Pepperoni Chaffles

**Preparation Time:** 5 minutes

**Cooking Time:** 5 Minutes

**Servings:** 2

**Ingredients:**

- 1 organic egg, beaten
- ½ cup Mozzarella cheese, shredded
- 2 tablespoons turkey pepperoni slice, chopped
- 1 tablespoon sugar-free pizza sauce
- ¼ teaspoon Italian seasoning

**Directions:**

1. Preheat a waffle iron and then grease it.
2. In a bowl, place all the ingredients and mix well.
3. Place the mixture into preheated waffle iron and cook for about 5 minutes or until golden brown.
4. Serve warm.

## Nutrition:

- Calories: 265
- Total Fat: 22g
- Protein: 13g
- Total Carbs: 8g
- Fiber: 3g
- Net Carbs: 5g
- Cholesterol: 121mg

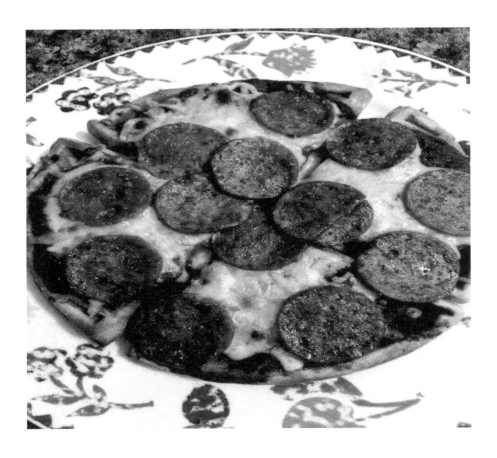

## 22.  Hot Sauce Jalapeño Chaffles

**Preparation Time:** 6 minutes

**Cooking Time:** 8 Minutes

**Servings:** 2

**Ingredients:**

- ½ cup plus 2 teaspoons Cheddar cheese, shredded and divided
- 1 organic egg, beaten
- 6 jalapeño pepper slices
- ¼ teaspoon hot sauce
- Pinch of salt

**Directions:**

1. Preheat a mini waffle iron and then grease it.
2. In a bowl, place ½ cup of cheese and remaining ingredients and mix until well combined.
3. Place about 1 teaspoon of cheese in the bottom of the waffle maker for about seconds before adding the mixture.
4. Place half of the mixture into preheated waffle iron and cook for about 3-minutes or until golden brown.
5. Repeat with the remaining cheese and mixture.
6. Serve warm.

## Nutrition:

- Calories: 336
- Total Fat: 28g
- Protein: 15g
- Total Carbs: 9g
- Fiber: 6g
- Net Carbs: 3g
- Cholesterol: 162mg

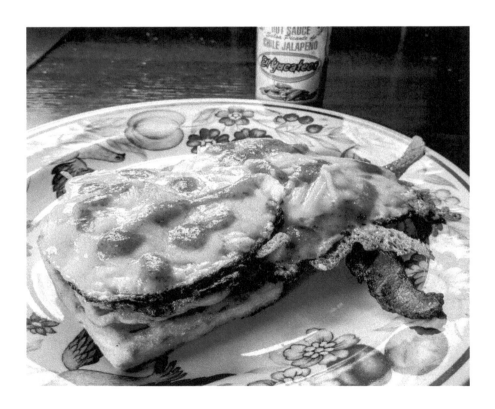

## 23. Chicken Chaffles

**Preparation Time:** 10 minutes

**Cooking Time:** 15 Minutes

**Servings:** 2

**Ingredients:**

- 2 oz chicken breasts, cooked, shredded
- 1/2 cup mozzarella cheese, finely shredded
- 2 eggs
- 6 tbsp parmesan cheese, finely shredded
- 1 cup zucchini, grated
- ½ cup almond flour
- 1tsp baking powder
- ¼ tsp garlic powder
- ¼ tsp black pepper, ground
- ½ tsp Italian seasoning
- ¼ tsp salt

**Directions:**

1. Sprinkle the zucchini with a pinch of salt and set it aside for a few minutes. Squeeze out the excess water.
2. Warm up your mini waffle maker.
3. Mix chicken, almond flour, baking powder, cheeses, garlic powder, salt, pepper and seasonings in a bowl.
4. Use another small bow for beating eggs. Add them to squeezed zucchini, mix well.
5. Combine the chicken and egg mixture, and mix.
6. For a crispy crust, add a teaspoon of shredded cheese to the waffle maker and cook for 30 seconds.
7. Then, pour the mixture into the waffle maker and cook for 5 minutes or until crispy.

8. Carefully remove. Repeat with remaining batter the same steps.
9. Enjoy!

## Nutrition:

- Calories: 341
- Total Fat: 27g
- Protein: 21g
- Total Carbs: 1g
- Fiber: 0g
- Net Carbs: 1g
- Cholesterol: 134mg

## 24. Garlicky Chicken Chaffles

**Preparation Time:** 6 minutes

**Cooking Time:** 12 Minutes

**Servings:** 2

**Ingredients:**

- 1 organic egg, beaten
- 1/3 cup grass-fed cooked chicken, chopped
- 1/3 cup Mozzarella cheese, shredded
- ¼ teaspoon garlic, minced
- ¼ teaspoon dried basil, crushed

**Directions:**

1. Preheat a mini waffle iron and then grease it.
2. In a bowl, place all the ingredients and mix until well combined.
3. Place half of the mixture into preheated waffle iron and cook for about 4-6 minutes or until golden brown.
4. Repeat with the remaining mixture.
5. Serve warm.

## Nutrition:

- Calories: 302
- Total Fat: 26g
- Protein: 13g
- Total Carbs: 5g
- Fiber: 2g Net
- Carbs: 3g
- Cholesterol: 320mg

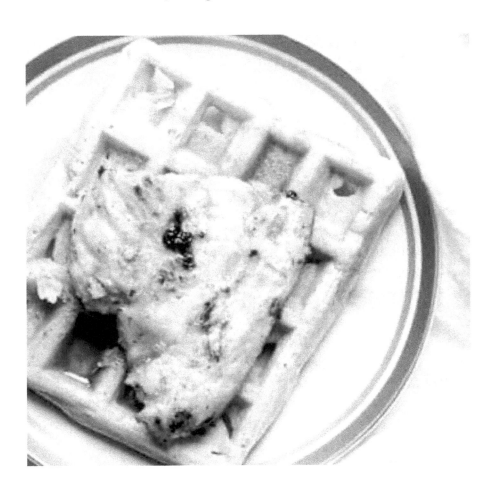

# SWEET CHAFFLE RECIPES

## 25. Blueberry Cream

**Preparation Time:** 10 minutes

**Cooking Time:** 8 minutes

**Servings:** 2

**Ingredients:**

- 1 organic egg, beaten
- 1 tablespoon cream cheese, softened
- 3 tablespoons almond flour
- ¼ teaspoon organic baking powder
- 1 teaspoon organic blueberry extract
- 5-6 fresh blueberries

**Directions:**

1. Preheat a mini waffle iron and then grease it.
2. In a bowl, place all the ingredients except blueberries and beat until well combined.
3. Fold in the blueberries.
4. Divide the mixture into 5 portions.
5. Place 1 portion of the mixture into preheated waffle iron and cooking for about 3-4 minutes or until golden brown.
6. Repeat with the remaining mixture.
7. Serve warm.

**Nutrition:**

- Calories: 160
- Protein: 7 g
- Carbohydrates: 4 g
- Fat: 3.5 g

## 26.   Strawberry Chaffles

**Preparation Time:** 10 minutes

**Cooking Time:** 8 minutes

**Servings:** 2

**Ingredients:**

- 1 organic egg, beaten
- ¼ cup Mozzarella cheese, shredded
- 1 tablespoon cream cheese, softened
- ¼ teaspoon organic baking powder
- 1 teaspoon organic strawberry extract
- 2 fresh strawberries, hulled and sliced

**Directions:**

1. Preheat a mini waffle iron and then grease it.
2. In a bowl, place all ingredients except strawberry slices and beat until well combined.
3. Fold in the strawberry slices.
4. Place half of the mixture into preheated waffle iron and cooking for about 4 minutes or until golden brown.
5. Repeat with the remaining mixture.
6. Serve warm.

**Nutrition:**

- Calories: 210
- Carbohydrates: 68 g
- Fat: 19 g
- Sugar: 39 g

# 27.  Berries Chaffles

**Preparation Time:** 10 minutes

**Cooking Time:** 10 minutes

**Servings:** 2

**Ingredients:**

- 1 organic egg
- 1 teaspoon organic vanilla extract
- 1 tablespoon of almond flour
- 1 teaspoon organic baking powder
- Pinch of ground cinnamon
- 1 cup Mozzarella cheese, shredded
- 2 tablespoons fresh blueberries
- 2 tablespoons fresh blackberries

**Directions:**

1. Preheat a waffle iron and then grease it.
2. In a bowl, place thee egg and vanilla extract and beat well.
3. Add the flour, baking powder and cinnamon and mix well.
4. Add the Mozzarella cheese and mix until just combined.
5. Gently, fold in the berries.
6. Place half of the mixture into preheated waffle iron and cooking for about 4-5 minutes or until golden brown.
7. Repeat with the remaining mixture.
8. Serve warm.

**Nutrition:**

- Calories: 200
- Fats: 1.5 g
- Carbohydrates: 23.4 g
- Fiber: 1.3 g

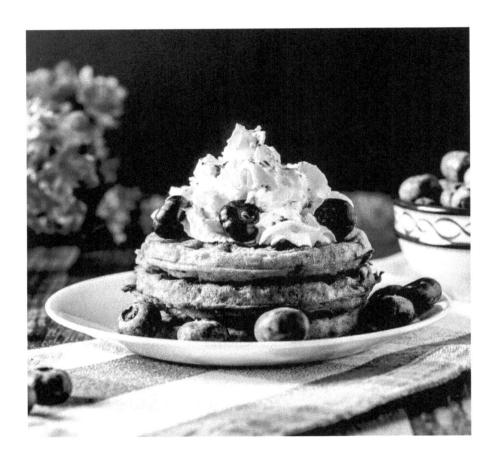

## 28. Coconut & Walnut Chaffle

**Preparation Time:** 10 minutes

**Cooking Time:** 24 minutes

**Servings:** 8

**Ingredients:**

- 4 organic eggs, beaten
- 4 ounces cream cheese, softened
- 1 tablespoon butter, melted
- 4 tablespoons coconut flour
- 1 tablespoon almond flour
- 2 tablespoons Erythritol
- 1½ teaspoons organic baking powder
- 1 teaspoon organic vanilla extract
- ½ teaspoon ground cinnamon
- 1 tablespoon unsweetened coconut, shredded
- 1 tablespoon walnuts, chopped

**Directions:**

- Preheat a mini waffle iron and then grease it.
- In a blender, place all ingredients and pulse until creamy and smooth.
- Divide the mixture into 8 portions.
- Place 1 portion of the mixture into preheated waffle iron and cooking for about 2-3 minutes or until golden brown.
- Repeat with the remaining mixture.
- Serve warm.

## Nutrition:

- Calories: 380
- Protein: 22 g
- Carbohydrates: 16 g

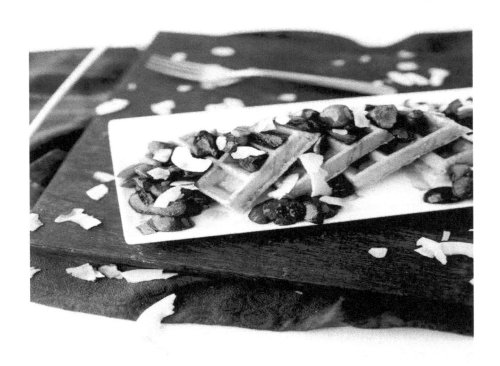

## 29.  Vanilla Raspberry Chaffle

**Preparation Time:** 5 minutes

**Cooking Time:** 8 minutes

**Servings:** 2

**Ingredients**

- ½ cup cream cheese, soft
- 1 teaspoon vanilla extract
- 1 tablespoon almond flour
- ¼ cup raspberries, pureed
- 1 egg, whisked
- 1 tablespoon monk fruit

**Directions**

1. In a bowl, mix the cream cheese with the raspberry puree and the other ingredients and whisk well.
2. Heat up the waffle iron over high heat, pour half of the batter, close the waffle maker, cooking for 8 minutes and transfer to a plate.
3. Repeat with the rest of the batter and servings the chaffles warm.

## Nutrition:

- Calories: 200
- Protein: 7 g
- Carbohydrates: 4 g
- Fat: 3.5 g

## 30. Pumpkin & Psyllium Husk Chaffles

**Preparation Time:** 8 minutes

**Cooking Time:** 16 Minutes

**Servings:** 2

**Ingredients:**

- 2 organic eggs
- ½ cup mozzarella cheese, shredded
- 1 tablespoon homemade pumpkin puree
- 2 teaspoons Erythritol
- ½ teaspoon psyllium husk powder
- 1/3 teaspoon ground cinnamon
- Pinch of salt
- ½ teaspoon organic vanilla extract

**Directions:**

1. Preheat a mini waffle iron and then grease it.
2. In a bowl, place all ingredients and beat until well combined.
3. Place ¼ of the mixture into preheated waffle iron and cook for about 4 minutes or until golden brown.
4. Repeat with the remaining mixture.
5. Serve warm.

## Nutrition:

- Calories: 400
- Carbohydrates: 51 g
- Fats: 5 g
- Fiber: 8 g

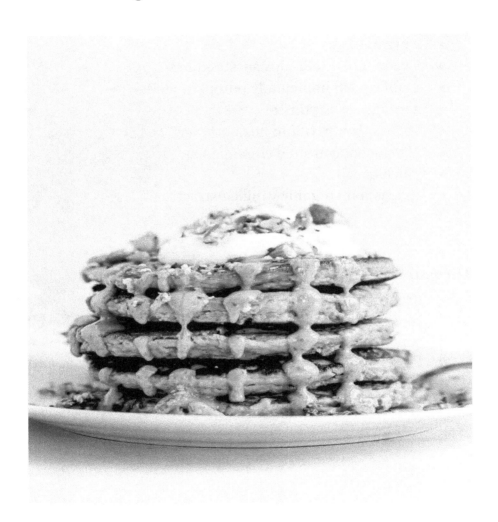

## 31. Blackberry Chaffles

**Preparation Time:** 5 minutes

**Cooking Time:** 8 Minutes

**Servings:** 2

**Ingredients:**

- 1 organic egg, beaten
- 1/3 cup Mozzarella cheese, shredded
- 1 teaspoon cream cheese, softened
- 1 teaspoon coconut flour
- ¼ teaspoon organic baking powder
- ¾ teaspoon powdered Erythritol
- ¼ teaspoon ground cinnamon
- ¼ teaspoon organic vanilla extract
- Pinch of salt
- 1 tablespoon fresh blackberries

**Directions:**

1. Preheat a mini waffle iron and then grease it.
2. In a bowl, place all ingredients except for blackberries and beat until well combined.
3. Fold in the blackberries.
4. Place half of the mixture into preheated waffle iron and cook for about minutes or until golden brown.
5. Repeat with the remaining mixture.
6. Serve warm.

## Nutrition:

- Calories: 360
- Fats: 1.5 g
- Protein: 49 g
- Carbohydrates: 40 g

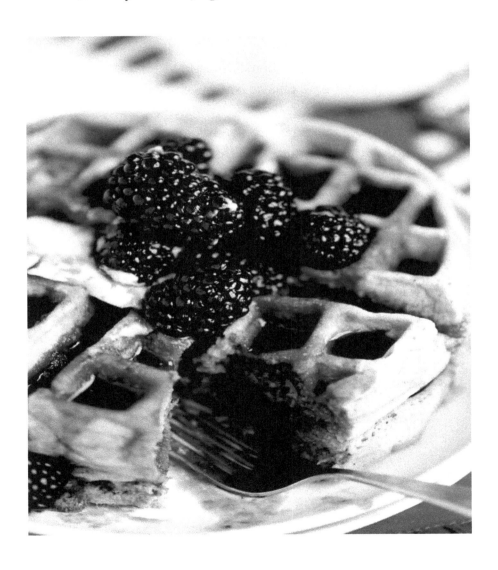

# 32. Cinnamon Pecan Chaffles

**Preparation Time:** 5 minutes

**Cooking Time:** 40 Minutes

**Servings:** 1

**Ingredients:**

- 1 Tbsp butter
- 1 egg
- ½ tsp vanilla
- 2 Tbsp almond flour
- 1 Tbsp coconut flour
- 1/8 tsp baking powder
- 1 Tbsp monk fruit
- For the crumble:
- ½ tsp cinnamon
- 1 Tbsp melted butter
- 1 tsp monk fruit
- 1 Tbsp chopped pecans

**Directions:**

1. Turn on waffle maker to heat and oil it with cooking spray.
2. Melt butter in a bowl, then mix in the egg and vanilla.
3. Mix in remaining chaffle ingredients.
4. Combine crumble ingredients in a separate bowl.
5. Pour half of the chaffle mix into waffle maker. Top with half of crumble mixture.
6. Cook for 5 minutes, or until done.
7. Repeat with the other half of the batter.

**Nutrition:**

- Carbs: g
- Fat: 35 g
- Protein: 10 g
- Calories: 391

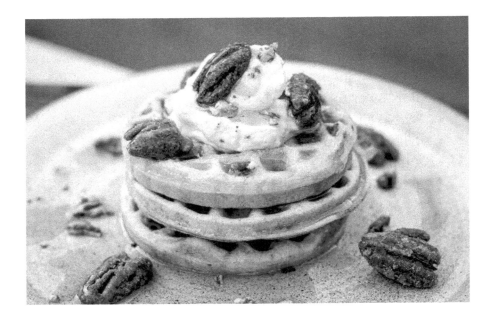

# MORE KETO CHAFFLE RECIPES

## 33. Coconut Oil Chaffles

**Preparation Time:** 6 minutes

**Cooking Time:** 5 minutes

**Servings:** 4

**Ingredients:**

- 1 tablespoon coconut oil, melted
- 1 cup almond flour
- 1 egg, whisked
- 3 tablespoons cream cheese, soft
- 1 and ½ cups almond milk
- 3 tablespoons stevia
- 2 tablespoons pumpkin seeds
- 1 teaspoon vanilla extract
- 1 teaspoon baking soda

**Directions:**

1. In a bowl, mix the melted coconut oil with the flour and the other ingredients and whisk well.
2. Heat up the waffle iron, pour ¼ of the batter and cooking for 5 minutes.
3. Repeat with the rest of the batter and serve the chaffles cold.

**Nutrition:**

- Total Fat 4g
- Calories 70
- Saturated Fat 1g
- Total Carbs 9g
- Net Carbs 7g
- Protein 1g
- Sugar: 4g
- Fiber 2g,
- Sodium 273mg
- Potassium 263mg

## 34. Almond and Nutmeg Chaffles

**Preparation Time:** 10 minutes

**Cooking Time:** 10 minutes

**Servings:** 6

**Ingredients:**

- 1 cup coconut flour
- ½ cup cream cheese, soft
- ½ teaspoon nutmeg, ground
- 1 cup almond flour
- 3 eggs, whisked
- ¼ cup almond butter, melted

**Directions:**

1. In a bowl, combine the flour with the cream cheese and the other ingredients and whisk.
2. Heat up the waffle iron, pour 1/6 of the batter and cooking for 7 minutes.
3. Repeat with the rest of the batter and serve.

**Nutrition:**

- Calories 53
- Total Fat 6g
- Saturated Fat 2g
- Total Carbs 2g
- Net Carbs 1g
- Protein 3g
- Sugar: 1g
- Fiber 1g
- Sodium 228mg
- Potassium 159mg

## 35. Lime Chaffles

**Preparation Time:** 10 minutes

**Cooking Time:** 10 minutes

**Servings:** 6

**Ingredients:**

- 1/3 cup almond butter, melted
- Juice and zest of 1 lime
- 1 cup almond flour
- ½ cup almond milk
- 3 tablespoons cream cheese, soft
- 1 egg, whisked
- 1 tablespoon stevia
- 1 and ½ tablespoons coconut oil

**Directions:**

1. In a bowl, combine the almond butter with the lime juice, zest and the other ingredients and whisk well.
2. Heat up the waffle iron, pour 1/6 of the batter inside and cooking for 7 minutes.
3. Repeat with the rest of the batter and serve the chaffles cold.

## Nutrition:

- Calories 83
- Total Fat 3g
- Saturated Fat 0.5g
- Total Carbs 14g
- Net Carbs 12g
- Protein 2g
- Sugar: 1g
- Fiber 2g
- Sodium 8mg
- Potassium 211mg

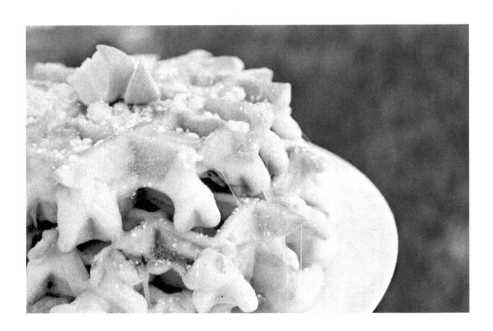

## 36. Blackberry and Cream Chaffles

**Preparation Time:** 10 minutes

**Cooking Time:** 10 minutes

**Servings:** 6

**Ingredients:**

- 1 and ¾ cup coconut flour
- Zest from 1 lime, grated
- ¼ cup blackberries
- ¼ cup cranberries
- 2 teaspoons baking powder
- ¼ cup swerve
- ¼ cup heavy cream
- ¼ cup cream cheese, warm
- 2 eggs, whisked
- 1 teaspoon vanilla extract

**Directions:**

1. In a bowl, mix the flour with the berries, lime zest and the other ingredients and whisk well.
2. Heat up the waffle iron, pour 1/6 of the batter and cooking for 8 minutes.
3. Repeat with the rest of the batter and serve.

**Nutrition:**

- Calories 64
- Fat 3.1 g
- Fiber 3 g
- Carbs 7.1 g
- Protein 2.8 g

## 37. Fruity Chaffles

**Preparation Time:** 10 minutes

**Cooking Time:** 10 minutes

**Servings:** 6

**Ingredients:**

- ½ cup almond flour
- ½ cup almond milk
- ½ cup coconut flour
- ½ cup cream cheese, soft
- 2 eggs, whisked
- 1 plum, pitted and chopped
- 1 avocado, peeled, pitted and chopped
- 1 mango, peeled, pitted and chopped
- ¼ teaspoon cinnamon, ground
- ½ teaspoon baking powder

**Directions:**

1. In your food processor, combine the flour with the milk, cream cheese and the other ingredients and pulse well.
2. Heat up the waffle iron over medium-high heat, pour 1/6 of the batter and cooking for 8 minutes.
3. Repeat with the rest of the batter and serve the chaffles cold.

## Nutrition:

- Calories 80
- Fat 2.5 g
- Fiber 3.9 g
- Carbs 10.9 g
- Protein 4 g

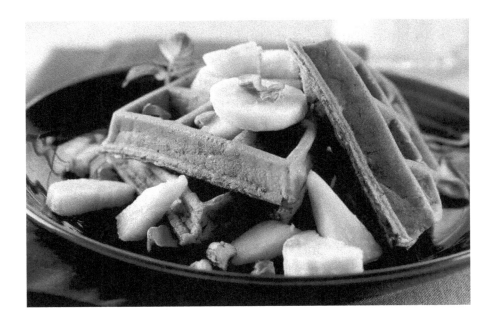

## 38.  Sweet Tomato Chaffles

**Preparation Time:** 5 minutes

**Cooking Time:** 8 minutes

**Servings:** 6

**Ingredients:**

- 1 cup almond flour
- 3 tablespoons tomato passata
- 1 cup cream cheese, soft
- 2 eggs, whisked
- 1 tablespoon stevia
- 1 teaspoon avocado oil
- ½ cup coconut cream
- 1 tablespoon coconut butter, melted

**Directions:**

1. In a bowl, combine the flour with the passata and the other ingredients and whisk well.
2. Pour 1/6 of the batter into the heated waffle maker and cooking for 8 minutes.
3. Repeat with the rest of the batter and serve.

## Nutrition:

- Calories 43
- Fat 3.4 g
- Fiber 1.7 g
- Carbs 3.4 g
- Protein 1.3 g

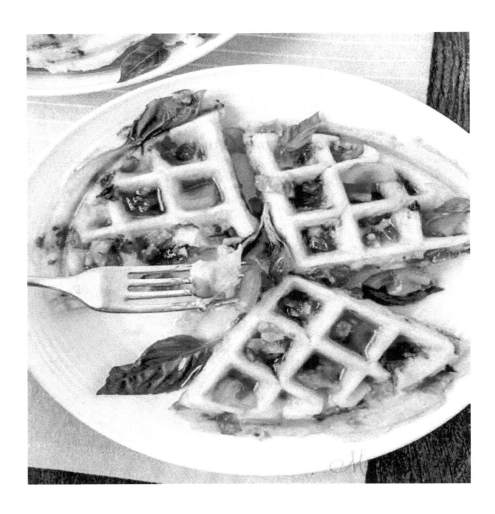

## 39. Delicious Milked Chaffles

**Preparation Time:** 5 minutes

**Cooking Time:** 10 minutes

**Servings:** 4

**Ingredients:**

- 1 tablespoon coconut oil, melted
- 1 and ½ cups almond milk
- 1 cup cauliflower rice
- 3 tablespoons stevia
- ½ cup almond flour
- ½ cup cream cheese, soft
- 1 egg, whisked
- 1 teaspoon vanilla extract
- 1 teaspoon baking soda

**Directions:**

1. In a bowl, mix the almond milk with the cauliflower rice and the other ingredients and whisk well.
2. Pour ¼ of the batter in the waffle iron, cooking for 8 minutes and transfer to a plate.
3. Repeat with the rest of the batter and serve the chaffles warm.

**Nutrition:**

- Calories 81
- Fat 4.2 g
- Fiber 6.5 g
- Carbs 11.1 g
- Protein 1.9 g

## 40. Mango and Berries Chaffles

**Preparation Time:** 10 minutes

**Cooking Time:** 10 minutes

**Servings:** 4

**Ingredients:**

- ½ cup mango, peeled and cubed
- 1 cup blueberries
- 1 cup almond flour
- ½ cup cream cheese, soft
- 2 eggs, whisked
- 1 tablespoon heavy cream
- 1 teaspoon baking powder
- 3 tablespoons cashew butter

**Directions:**

1. In a bowl, combine the mango with the berries and the other ingredients and whisk well.
2. Pour ¼ of the batter in the waffle iron, cooking for 7 minutes and transfer to a plate.
3. Repeat with the rest of the batter and serve the chaffles warm.

## Nutrition:

- Calories 526
- Fat 53.2 g
- Fiber 7.8 g
- Carbs 11.7 g
- Protein 8.2 g

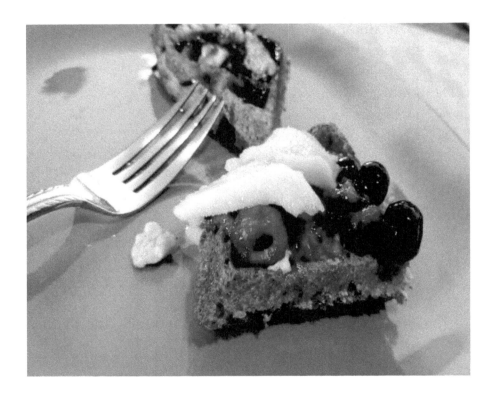

# CONCLUSION

Chaffles is the amazing new invention you've been waiting for. It's a revolutionary, patent-pending, and 100% vegan protein bar with a thousand uses.

What are chaffles? Chaffles is a delicious new product that can be used to replace the high fat and high sugar snacks in your diet like cheese chips or chocolate bars. It's also gluten-free, vegan, non-GMO, low in sodium and preservative free! The best part is that chaffles taste just as good as candy! You'll never want anything else again after trying this life changing snack.

The combination of protein and savory chaffle taste will keep you wanting to eat more every time. Chaffles are also a great substitute for those times that you feel like having something sweet, but want something healthy with a lot of flavor.

Chaffles come in an assortment of flavors like Pecan Pie or Cherry Pie and can be served with a drizzle of your favorite nut butter or cinnamon sugar for an awesome snack. Or you can create your own combinations by mixing them up the way that makes your mouth water.

Chaffles are great for both kids and adults. They're the perfect snack to bring on a hike for an afternoon treat or to eat on a road trip or flights. Even better, they create a new way for parents to get their kids to eat protein without them even knowing what they're eating. Now if you want your children to enjoy healthy food without complaining, chaffles will be your best friend.

No matter what you eat chaffles with, it will never disappoint! Have it with chicken noodle soup or mashed potatoes for dinner or have it with salad at lunch.

Chaffle is a perfect combination for keto dieters. Besides, keto diet is always low in carbs and high in fat so chaffle is an amazing option for it.

Chaffles are very versatile and can be used as a spread for your favorite bagel or toast, or even on top of a pizza before baking it. You can also use chaffles as an ingredient for your own meals like pancakes, pies, donuts, breads and so much more!

Chaffle comes in two different flavors: savory and sweet. The savory flavor is more of a BBQ flavor while the sweet flavor is more cookie dough style. The savory chaffles are perfect for replacing things like bread and crackers, while sweet chaffles can be used as a dessert or drink! You can also add chaffle to your favorite dessert recipes for an amazing taste.

Chaffles are the most unique tasting protein bar around that is also good for you. You won't believe how good they taste until you try them for yourself. This incredible product is sure to revolutionize your snacking experience and change the way you think about eating healthy forever.

Always remember when making your own chaffle recipes, you can choose from almost any combination of things like fruits, cereals, nuts and seeds. You can even use different types of chocolate in some recipes. Anything goes with chaffle!

What's even more exciting is that chaffles come in many sizes to fit anyone's taste and diet.

It's time to ditch your unhealthy snacks for life changing chaffles!

CPSIA information can be obtained
at www.ICGtesting.com
Printed in the USA
BVHW090326220621
610126BV00012B/2901